REFLEXOLOGY

MANUAL

Unlocking Natural Healing, Comprehensive Guide To Reflexology Techniques, Zones, Stress Relief, Pain Management, And Holistic Wellness

LAMBERT FETTERMAN

DISCLAIMER

The content in this book is offered only for general informative purposes. While every effort has been taken to guarantee the content's accuracy and completeness, the author and publisher accept no responsibility for any mistakes or omissions, or for the results of using the information given herein. The methods, recommendations, and directions in this book are not guaranteed to be appropriate for every person, and readers should exercise caution and seek professional counsel if required before undertaking any of the projects or techniques detailed in this book.

Table of Contents

INTRODUCTION

Reflexology is a holistic therapeutic technique that includes applying pressure to certain spots on the feet, hands, or ears to promote healing and relieve a variety of health problems across the body.

Understanding Reflexology

Reflexology is a holistic treatment therapy that includes applying pressure to particular spots on the feet, hands, or ears to enhance general health and balance. The concept that these precise sites, known as reflex points, relate to distinct organs, glands, and systems in the body is at the heart of reflexology. Practitioners hope to ease stress, tension, and imbalances by activating these reflex spots, hence boosting the body's natural healing processes.

Reflexology is based on ancient Chinese and Egyptian techniques, with historical evidence extending back thousands of years. These civilizations believed in energy routes throughout the body, and reflexology emerged as a method of balancing and harmonizing these energies. Reflexology has incorporated components from numerous therapeutic systems, including Chinese medicine, zone treatment, and Native American healing methods, throughout time.

History And Origins

Reflexology may be traced back to ancient cultures when foot and hand remedies were used for healing. The Chinese are credited with pioneering foot treatment, with their knowledge of energy movement in the body influenced by the notion of Qi and meridians. Pressure on the foot was also used in ancient Egyptian traditions to aid healing.

A kind of zone treatment, a forerunner of reflexology, originated in the United States in the early twentieth century. Dr. William H. Fitzgerald, an ear, nose, and throat specialist, proposed that the body may be split into 10 longitudinal zones, each corresponding to a different finger or toe.

This paved the way for contemporary reflexology.

In the 1930s, physiotherapist Eunice Ingham expanded on reflexology. She created the reflexology charts that are now widely used by mapping the complete body on the feet and hands. Ingham's work was crucial in the expansion and acceptance of reflexology as a treatment.

Today, reflexology is widely accepted as a supplementary treatment, often utilized in combination with traditional medicine. Its vast history and numerous cultural influences make it a fascinating and ever-changing subject of holistic treatment.

CHAPTER 1

Principles Of Reflexology

Fundamentals Of Reflex Zones

Reflexology assumes that the body is replicated in miniature on the feet, hands, and ears via reflex zones or points. These reflex zones relate to certain physical locations, organs, or systems. For example, the tip of the big toe may symbolize the head, while the heel may represent the lower back or pelvic region.

These zones are said to be linked by energy channels, allowing energy or life force to move throughout the body. Practitioners want to achieve equilibrium and stimulate the body's natural healing processes by triggering these reflexes.

How Reflexology Works

Pressure is applied to these sensitive zones utilizing specialized thumb, finger, and hand methods in reflexology procedures. Practitioners hope to relieve stress, increase circulation, and promote general relaxation by stimulating these spots. Pressure is thought to deliver relaxing signals to the neurological system, helping the body to restore equilibrium and improve well-being.

Connection To The Nervous System

The efficiency of reflexology is linked to its impact on the neurological system. Reflex point stimulation causes nerve responses that correlate to particular locations of the body. This stimulation is thought to create a neurological pathway that urges the body to react, relax, and perhaps reduce pain or imbalances in the affected regions.

Understanding these essential concepts serves as the foundation for reflexology practice, assisting practitioners in locating and activating reflex zones to promote well-being and support the body's natural healing processes.

CHAPTER 2

Mapping The Body Through Feet And Hands

Reflexology is a holistic treatment in which pressure is applied to certain areas on the feet and hands to promote relaxation, balance, and general well-being. Understanding the body map via the feet and hands is essential to the practice. This chapter delves into the detailed features of these extremities' reflex zones and their relationship to numerous bodily organs and systems.

Reflex Areas On The Feet

In reflexology, the feet function as a microcosm of the whole body. Practitioners may discover locations that correlate to particular organs, glands, and bodily components by separating the foot into distinct zones and sections. The reflex zones of the foot are linked by energy channels, illustrating the idea that the body is a single organism.

1. **Toes:** The tips of the toes are linked to the skull, which includes the brain and sinuses. Massage and pressure on this region may help relieve headaches and nasal congestion.

2. The ball of the foot connects to the heart and chest. It is often used to promote cardiovascular health and alleviate respiratory difficulties.

3. The digestive system is represented by the middle arch of the foot. Working on this region may assist in digestion and the

treatment of stomach and intestinal problems.

4. Heel: The foot's heel is connected to the lower back and pelvic area. Lower back pain and stiffness may be relieved with reflexology in this region.

5. The spine (inner edge) and the shoulders and limbs (outer edge) are represented by these edges. Addressing these issues may help to improve spinal health and general muscle well-being.

Reflex Areas On The Hands

While reflexology is often linked with the feet, the hands play an important part in this therapy as well. The reflex zones on the hands and feet mirror each other, providing an alternate or complementary method for managing a variety of health conditions.

1. Fingers: The fingers, like the toes, are related to the head. Each finger represents a different location, with the thumb representing the brain and the index finger representing the sinuses.

2. Thumb: Because the thumb reflects the head and neck, it is an important region to relieve tension and promote relaxation in these areas.

3. The digestive organs are represented by the center area of the palm. Practitioners hope to improve gut health by focusing on this region.

4. The base of the thumb is connected to the neck and thyroid gland. Individuals suffering from neck stress or thyroid problems may benefit from reflexology in this area.

5. Heel of the Hand: The pelvic area is represented by the heel of the hand. Reflexology in this region may be utilized to treat reproductive system and lower back problems.

Correspondence To Body Organs And Systems

Recognizing the relationship of reflex zones on the feet and hands to certain bodily organs and systems is necessary for understanding them.

Reflexology charts, which represent the link between these zones and the rest of the body, are often used as visual aids.

1. Endocrine System: Endocrine glands, such as the pituitary gland, thyroid gland, and adrenal glands, are related to points on the inside of the feet and hands. Balancing these points may help with hormonal equilibrium.

2. Digestive System: The stomach, liver, gallbladder, and intestines are represented by reflex zones on the center section of the feet and hands. The goal of stimulating these regions is to improve digestion and nutrition absorption.

3. Cardiovascular System: Because the ball of the foot resembles the heart, reflexology

in this region is said to benefit heart health and circulation.

4. Respiratory System: Because reflex points on the toes and fingers are related to the respiratory system, they are important regions for treating breathing problems and boosting lung health.

5. The musculoskeletal system, which includes the spine and limbs, is represented by the outside borders of the feet and hands. In these places, reflexology may help reduce stress and increase flexibility.

In conclusion, mapping the body via the feet and hands is a fundamental component of reflexology. This information is used by practitioners to personalize their approach to individual requirements, encouraging balance and energy throughout the body. This awareness of the body's reflex zones serves as the foundation for successful and focused practice as we continue our research of reflexology.

CHAPTER 3

Techniques And Tools

Reflexology Techniques

Reflexology uses a variety of ways to activate reflex sites. Thumb walking is a common technique in which moderate pressure is given over the foot or hand with the thumb in a walking motion. Depending on the reflexologist's technique and the individual's demands, rotational motions and kneading may also be employed.

Variations In Pressure And Strokes

The amount of pressure used during reflexology varies based on the individual's degree of comfort and the region being worked on. For delicate locations, utilize gentle pressure, whereas deeper reflex sites need greater pressure. Strokes may also vary, from circular to linear, with each aiming to activate the relevant reflex zone.

Introduction To Tools (E.G., Charts, Rollers)

Reflexology instruments, including charts and rollers, may help to improve the practice. Reflexology charts vividly map out the reflex points on the feet and hands, guiding practitioners and self-reflexologists alike. Rollers, which are often constructed of wood or metal, may be used to provide regulated pressure to certain reflex zones, assisting in both relaxation and stimulation of these regions.

Reflexologists use these methods and instruments to induce relaxation, increase circulation, and perhaps reduce pain or imbalances in the body. Understanding how to properly utilize these strategies is critical in the practice of reflexology.

CHAPTER 4

Reflexology And Health Benefits

Stress Relief And Relaxation

One of reflexology's key advantages is its ability to create relaxation and ease tension. Reflexology treatments stimulate the nervous system, encouraging relaxation reactions inside the body. Reflexology helps release endorphins, which calms the mind and body by targeting reflex spots, particularly those related to stress and tension. This relaxation technique helps to alleviate stress-related symptoms such as anxiety, tension headaches, and sleep difficulties.

Improving Circulation

Reflexology has been shown to improve blood circulation throughout the body. It increases blood flow to many organs and systems by applying pressure to reflex sites. This enhanced circulation not only improves the delivery of oxygen and minerals but also assists in the elimination of toxins and metabolic waste from the tissues. It helps to maintain good health by supporting the entire function of the cardiovascular system.

Enhancing Overall Well-Being

Reflexology aids in overall well-being in addition to stress reduction and increased circulation. The practice aids the body's natural healing processes by activating the nervous system and establishing internal harmony. Reflexology, by concentrating on certain reflex points, helps to restore harmony to the relevant organs and systems, creating a feeling of general health and wholeness.

Reflexology's effectiveness in increasing relaxation, circulation, and general well-being has been recognized in alternative medicine. Its non-invasive nature and possible advantages for a variety of health issues make it a popular option among those looking for natural treatment approaches.

Understanding the tremendous effect reflexology may have on the body lays the groundwork for investigating its use in holistic health and wellness, which offers potential pathways for enhanced health and quality of life.

CHAPTER 5

Reflexology For Specific Conditions

Reflexology, as an alternative treatment, has the potential to address a variety of particular health conditions. Here's a more in-depth look:

Headaches And Migraines

Reflexologists often concentrate on particular locations connected to headaches and migraines. For example, stimulating the toes or the sides of the feet is said to help with headache alleviation. The notion is based on applying pressure to reflex spots on the head, neck, and shoulders to improve blood circulation and relieve stress.

The goal of reflexology is to stimulate the body's natural healing processes and minimize the frequency or severity of headaches.

Digestive Disorders

Reflexology treats digestive difficulties by focusing on reflex sites associated with the digestive system, such as the stomach, intestines, and liver. Practitioners hope to promote improved digestion, ease bloating, reduce pain, and help in the overall functioning of the digestive system by stimulating specific areas on the feet or hands. The pressure given to certain zones is said to promote relaxation and encourage the body to restore digestive system homeostasis.

Pain Management

Reflexology is now being researched as a supplemental way of pain management, particularly for chronic pain disorders. Practitioners want to trigger the body's natural pain-relief processes by concentrating on reflex points associated with regions of discomfort. It is thought that by applying pressure to certain zones, reflexology may cause the release of endorphins, the body's natural painkillers, so relieving pain and promoting relaxation.

The Holistic Method

Treating particular ailments is often part of a greater holistic approach in reflexology. Practitioners stress that the body is interrelated and that treating one region may have a good influence on other physiological systems. While reflexology seeks to address particular issues, the overarching objective is to restore balance and promote the body's inherent healing processes.

Reflexology As An Alternative Therapy

While reflexology may be beneficial, it is normally used in conjunction with other medical therapies. Many individuals appreciate reflexology as a complementary technique to controlling specific health concerns and include it in their wellness regimens. However, before utilizing reflexology as a single therapy for any medical ailment, it is critical to speak with a healthcare expert.

The potential of reflexology for certain illnesses is still being researched and pursued in the domain of alternative medicines. As practitioners improve their reflexology methods and knowledge, its uses for diverse health conditions may expand.

CHAPTER 6

Reflexology And Holistic Wellness

Integration With Other Healing Practices

Because reflexology is a holistic treatment, it often combines with other therapeutic approaches. It enhances the efficacy of techniques such as aromatherapy, acupuncture, and yoga. The combination of these methods fosters overall well-being by concurrently treating physical, mental, and emotional elements.

Complementary Therapies

Reflexology is seldom used alone; it is often coupled with other holistic therapies. When used with massage treatment, for example, the combination may induce a deep relaxation response that benefits both the body and the mind. Similarly, when combined with chiropractic therapy, reflexology helps to balance the body's energy flow.

Mind-Body Connection

The concept behind reflexology is based on the notion that the mind and body are inextricably linked. The body's innate healing systems are stimulated by activating reflex spots, affecting not just physical health but also mental and emotional well-being. The procedure may cause relaxation responses, reducing tension and anxiety and enhancing mental clarity.

Reflexology aids in the restoration of the body's equilibrium, cleansing, circulation improvement, and general vigor in holistic well-being. Furthermore, it is valued for its capacity to harmonize the mind and body, generating a feeling of harmony and balance.

This chapter dives into reflexology's collaborative character within the larger spectrum of holistic treatments, stressing its role in fostering overall well-being and balance across different aspects of health.

CHAPTER 7

Reflexology In Practice

Reflexology is a hands-on treatment that includes a systematic method and sensitivity to individual requirements. Here's a detailed look at the practical aspects:

Preparing For A Reflexology Session

1. Setting Up the Environment: Creating a Relaxing Atmosphere

• *Ambiance:* Creating a peaceful, pleasant atmosphere with soft lighting, comfy seats, and soothing music.

- *Cleanliness:* Maintaining hygiene via the use of clean towels, sterilized hands, and neat instruments or equipment.

2. Client Interaction and Evaluation

- *Intake Discussion:* Learn about the client's health history, issues, and session objectives.

- *Evaluation:* Examining the feet or hands for anomalies, sensitivities, or areas of pain.

3. Tools and Technique

- *Pressure Application:* Applying moderate pressure to reflex spots using the thumbs, fingers, or specialized equipment.

- *Strokes and Movements:* For stimulation, use varied strokes such as thumb-walking, rotation, or kneading.

• *Use of Oils or Lotions:* Some practitioners use natural oils to help with smoother motions and relaxation.

Conducting A Session Step-By-Step

1. Warm-Up Methods

• *Relaxation Techniques:* Using relaxation techniques such as deep breathing or relaxation exercises to help the client relax.

2. Methodical Approach

• *Mapping the Reflex Zones:* Addressing particular reflex zones about organs or systems systematically.

- *Focused Attention:* Consistently applying pressure to specific zones, progressively altering intensity depending on client input.

3. Observation and Reaction

- *Client Feedback:* Encourage clients to express any feelings, discomfort, or changes they experience throughout the session.

- *Adjusting Technique:* Changing pressure or technique based on the client's comfort level and reflex responses.

Addressing Client Concerns And Expectations

1. Communication
- *Process Explanation:* Provide an outline of what to anticipate during and after the session.

- *Managing Expectations:* Informing clients about possible post-session emotions or impacts.

2. After-Session Care

- Hydration: Encourage clients to drink water to flush out toxins and rehydrate themselves.

- *Recommendations for Follow-Up:* Advice on rest or other recommended self-care practices.

3. Client Participation

- *Comments and Follow-Up:* Welcoming comments to enhance future sessions, as well as considering the prospect of regular sessions for overall benefits.

Because reflexology isn't a one-size-fits-all approach, adaptation, attention, and client-centered care are essential for effective sessions. It is about providing a calm environment, recognizing the requirements of the person, and using well-practiced methods to promote relaxation and well-being.

CHAPTER 8

Reflexology Across Cultures

Reflexology In Traditional Medicine

1. Cultural Heritage: Reflexology is more than simply a current health fad; it has profound origins in many ancient healing systems across the world. Ancient Chinese medicine, Egyptian traditions, Native American healing procedures, and even Ayurveda in India are examples of this. Each culture evolved its reflexology technique, incorporating local beliefs, anatomy, and therapeutic concepts.

2.	Ancient Chinese Reflexology: Reflexology was included in Traditional Chinese Medicine (TCM) in China. It is similar to acupuncture and acupressure in that it is based on the notion of meridians and energy flow. To balance the body's Qi, the technique in China concentrates on precise pressure spots connected to meridians and essential energy flow.

3. Egyptian Influence: Foot massage and pressure points were used in ancient Egypt for therapeutic causes. Hieroglyphs portray images of foot and hand manipulation, implying a belief in reflexology's therapeutic abilities.

4. Native American Traditions: Reflexology was used by several Native American cultures, with pressure points on the feet or hands used to heal diseases and preserve well-being. Their approaches were based on the concept that nature, spirituality, and the human body were all interrelated.

Cultural Variations And Practices

1. Techniques and Methods: Reflexology treatments differ greatly among countries. Some cultures value the feet more than the hands, while others emphasize both the hands and the feet. Pressure application, massage methods, and belief in distinct response zones associated with bodily systems may vary amongst techniques.

2.   Ritual & Ceremony: Reflexology is considered a ritualistic or ceremonial activity in many cultures. It often combines with spiritual beliefs, employing medicines, oils, chants, or prayers to boost therapeutic results.

3.   Adaptation & Integration: Reflexology has crossed continents and adapted to many cultural situations. Modern reflexology practitioners sometimes combine methods from several traditions, combining knowledge and practices for a more holistic approach.

Understanding reflexology's rich history and many cultural adaptations not only emphasizes its universality but also improves its practice by embracing other ideas and methodologies, stressing the interdependence of human civilizations in the search for health and healing.

CHAPTER 9

Reflexology: Ethics And Professionalism

Like other holistic treatments, reflexology requires a delicate connection between the practitioner and the patient. Understanding the ethical framework and being professional are essential components of offering excellent reflexology treatments.

Code Of Conduct

Ethical principles are the foundation of reflexology work. They cover a wide range of topics, including confidentiality, respect, and the client's well-being. Adherence to a stringent code of conduct guarantees that the practitioner retains professionalism while also upholding the therapy's credibility.

1. Confidentiality: It is critical to respect customers' privacy and confidentiality. Unless otherwise agreed, information discussed during sessions should be kept secret.

2. Respect and decency: Practitioners must treat clients with decency and empathy, creating a welcoming and non-discriminatory workplace.

3. Informed Consent: Practitioners should describe the technique, its advantages, and any possible dangers or discomforts associated before the session. Before beginning therapy, acquire consent from the patient.

4. Professional Boundaries: It is critical to maintain professional boundaries. Practitioners must avoid any conduct that might be seen as disrespectful or unprofessional.

5. Continual Development: It is critical to commit to continual education and development. Practitioners must keep up to speed on new methods, research, and ethical norms in the profession.

Practitioner-Patient Relationship

It is critical to establish a good connection and create trust between the practitioner and the client.

Mutual respect, understanding, and open communication should underpin the connection.

1. Listening and communication: Understanding the client's demands requires active listening. Setting expectations and ensuring the customer feels heard and appreciated are aided by clear communication.

2. Empathy and Compassion: Practitioners should approach clients with empathy and compassion, listening to their issues and giving emotional support in addition to therapy.

3. Professional Integrity: Maintaining professional integrity entails acting ethically

and prioritizing client interests above personal benefit.

Continuing Education And Development

Reflexology is a growing subject, with new studies and methods being developed regularly. Practitioners must keep current on new advances to deliver the best possible treatment to their customers.

1. Continuous Learning: Participating in continual education and training helps practitioners enhance their abilities and keep up to date with reflexology advances.

2. Participation in seminars, workshops, and professional networks helps practitioners to

share information and experiences, building a supportive community within the area.

3. Compliance with legal rules and regulations ensures that practitioners maintain professional standards and work within the law.

Following ethical norms and being professional in reflexology practice not only provides excellent service but also increases the practitioner's reputation and reliability within the healthcare community.

CHAPTER 10

Reflexology: Future Trends And Advancements

Research And Scientific Studies

The advancement of reflexology is dependent on continual research to prove its usefulness. Researching the effect of reflex sites on health issues, the nervous system's reaction and plausible physiological causes might help influence future practices.

Innovations In Reflexology

Technological advancements, such as specialized instruments for more accuracy or data-driven techniques for individualized sessions, may supplement reflexology. The use of technology in reflexology methods might provide new insights or enhance therapeutic results.

Emerging Applications And Directions

Exploring novel reflexology uses, such as its incorporation into contemporary healthcare settings, may have a big influence on its awareness and acceptability. Furthering the development of reflexology for certain populations or illnesses may result in novel treatment techniques.

Cultural Adaptation And Integration

Because reflexology is used throughout cultures, knowing and incorporating different methods and ideologies may widen its reach. Exploring traditional methods from throughout the globe may provide reflexology with new views.

Complementary Medicine And Holistic Healthcare

The potential of reflexology in holistic health may continue to grow, particularly in integrative healthcare approaches. Collaborations with mainstream medicine or other alternative treatments may provide a more holistic approach to patient care.

Standardization And Education

Continued attempts to standardize reflexology procedures, create certification, and provide excellent education will help to boost its legitimacy. Collaboration with academic institutions and healthcare groups may be required.

Public Acceptance And Awareness

Increasing public knowledge via activism, scientific dissemination, and patient testimonies may aid in the acknowledgment and acceptance of reflexology within mainstream healthcare.

Accessibility And Sustainability

Making reflexology more accessible and affordable for various groups, such as underprivileged communities or distant places, has the potential to broaden its reach and influence.

Practice Based On Evidence

Reflexology's standing as a recognized therapeutic intervention may be strengthened by emphasizing evidence-based techniques via clinical trials, case studies, and recorded results.

Professional Development And Regulation

Advocating for clearer legislation, ethical norms, and professional development opportunities may help to raise the standards of reflexology practice, assuring both practitioner and client safety and quality.

Reflexology's development is characterized by an interdisciplinary approach that incorporates scientific findings, cultural insights, technology breakthroughs, and ethical issues. Keeping an eye on these future developments may help influence its expansion and integration into mainstream healthcare systems, maintaining its relevance and effectiveness in the years ahead.

Conclusion

The relevance of reflexology in contemporary health is varied. It complements traditional treatment as an alternative therapy by fostering overall well-being. The practice's capacity to trigger reflex zones on the feet and hands, hence promoting bodily harmony, is consistent with modern wellness ideas.

One critical feature is its incorporation into a holistic healthcare strategy. Reflexology is becoming more widely accepted in healthcare systems across the globe, serving as a supplement to standard therapies. Its non-invasive nature, as well as its focus on relaxation and stress reduction, contribute to patients' favorable experiences.

Furthermore, continued research into the mechanics and consequences of reflexology is critical. Scientific research is constantly being conducted to investigate the influence of reflexology on different illnesses, revealing information on its possible therapeutic uses. Such a study helps to verify and improve the status of reflexology in healthcare settings.

The importance of ethics and professionalism in enhancing the legitimacy of reflexology cannot be overstated. A strong code of conduct guarantees that practitioners maintain high standards of practice, which fosters confidence in the treatment. Respectful practitioner-patient relationships value patient comfort, confidentiality, and informed consent.

Reflexology practitioners must maintain their education and growth. Keeping up with advances in the industry improves their abilities and ensures the administration of safe and effective therapies. Collaboration with other healthcare specialists promotes an integrated approach, recognizing the role of reflexology in holistic therapy.

Finally, reflexology's evolution from ancient methods to current acceptability in healthcare demonstrates its ongoing importance. Encouragement of further study, research, and ethical practice will help cement reflexology's status as a vital component of holistic well-being, embracing tradition while enhancing its role in modern health.

THE END